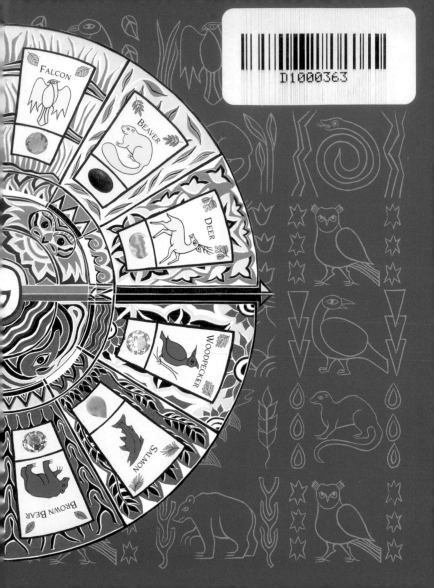

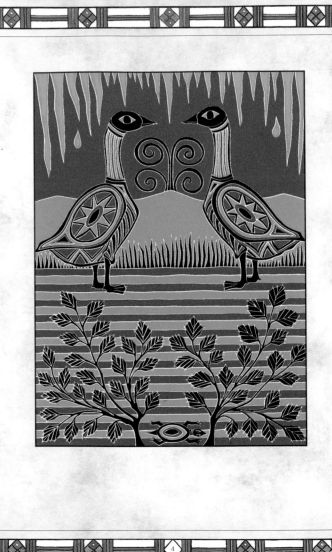

THE LITTLE LIBRARY OF
EARTH MEDICINE

GOOSE

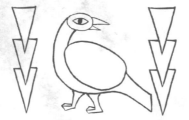

Kenneth Meadows
Illustrations by Jo Donegan

DORLING KINDERSLEY
LONDON • NEW YORK • SYDNEY • MOSCOW

A DORLING KINDERSLEY BOOK

Managing editor: Jonathan Metcalf
Managing art editor: Peter Cross
Production manager: Michelle Thomas

The Little Library of Earth Medicine was
produced, edited and designed by
GLS Editorial and Design
Garden Studios, 11-15 Betterton Street
London WC2H 9BP

GLS Editorial and Design
Editorial director: Jane Laing
Design director: Ruth Shane
Project designer: Luke Herriott
Editors: Claire Calman, Terry Burrows, Victoria Sorzano

Additional illustrations: Roy Flooks 16, 17, 31; John Lawrence 38
Special photography: Mark Hamilton
Picture credits: American Natural History Museum 8-9, 12, 14-15, 32

First published in Great Britain in 1998
by Dorling Kindersley Limited
9 Henrietta Street, London WC2E 8PS

2 4 6 8 10 9 7 5 3 1

A CIP catalogue record for this book is available from the British Library

UK ISBN 0 7513 0523 5   AUSTRALIAN ISBN 1 86466 040 6

Reproduced by Kestrel Digital Colour Ltd, Chelmsford, Essex
Printed and bound in Hong Kong by Imago

CONTENTS

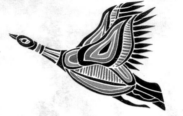

INTRODUCING
EARTH MEDICINE

TO NATIVE AMERICANS, MEDICINE IS NOT AN EXTERNAL SUBSTANCE BUT AN INNER POWER THAT IS FOUND IN BOTH NATURE AND OURSELVES.

E arth Medicine is a unique method of personality profiling that draws on Native American under-standing of the Universe, and on the principles embodied in sacred Medicine Wheels.

Native Americans believed that spirit, although invisible, permeated Nature, so that everything in Nature was sacred. Animals were perceived as acting as

messengers of spirit. They also appeared in waking dreams to impart power known as "medicine". The recipients of such dreams honoured the animal species that appeared to them by rendering their images on ceremonial and everyday artefacts.

NATURE WITHIN SELF

Native American shamans – tribal wisemen – recognized similarities between the natural forces prevalent during the seasons and the characteristics of those born

Shaman's rattle
Shamans used rattles to connect with their inner spirit. This is a Tlingit shaman's wooden rattle.

"Spirit has provided you with an opportunity to study in Nature's university." *Stoney teaching*

during corresponding times of the year. They also noted how personality is affected by the four phases of the Moon – at birth and throughout life – and by the continual alternation of energy flow, from active to passive. This view is encapsulated in Earth Medicine, which helps you to recognize how the dynamics of Nature function within you and how the potential strengths you were born with can be developed.

Animal ornament

To the Anasazi, who carved this ornament from jet, the frog symbolized adaptability.

MEDICINE WHEELS

Native American cultural traditions embrace a variety of circular symbolic images and objects. These sacred hoops have become known as Medicine

Wheels, due to their similarity to the spoked wheels of the wagons that carried settlers into the heartlands of once-Native American territory. Each Medicine Wheel showed how different objects or qualities related to one another within the context of a greater whole, and how different forces and energies moved within it.

One Medicine Wheel might be regarded as the master wheel because it indicated balance within Nature and the most effective way of achieving harmony with the Universe and ourselves. It is upon this master Medicine Wheel (see pp.10–11) that Earth Medicine is structured.

Feast dish

Stylized bear carvings adorn this Tlingit feast dish. To the American Indian, the bear symbolizes strength and self-sufficiency.

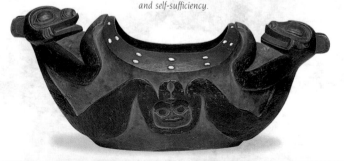

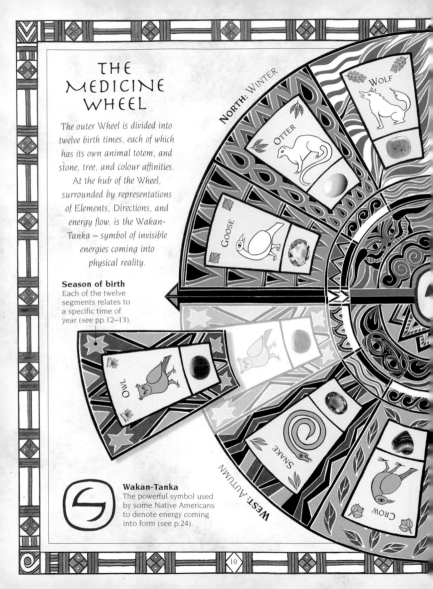

THE MEDICINE WHEEL

The outer Wheel is divided into twelve birth times, each of which has its own animal totem, and stone, tree, and colour affinities. At the hub of the Wheel, surrounded by representations of Elements, Directions, and energy flow, is the Wakan-Tanka – symbol of invisible energies coming into physical reality.

Season of birth
Each of the twelve segments relates to a specific time of year (see pp.12–13).

Wakan-Tanka
The powerful symbol used by some Native Americans to denote energy coming into form (see p.24).

NORTH: WINTER

WEST: AUTUMN

WOLF

OTTER

GOOSE

OWL

SNAKE

CROW

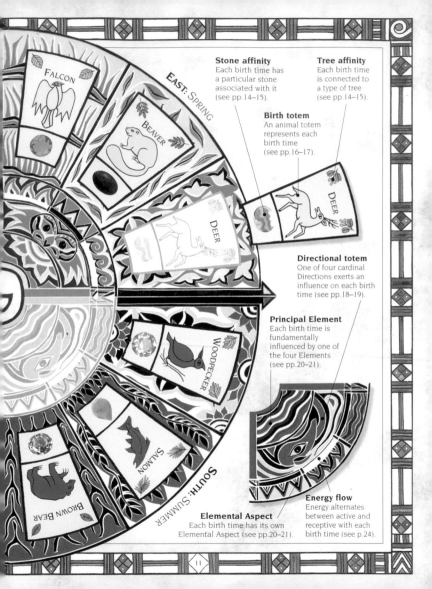

EAST: SPRING

FALCON

BEAVER

DEER

DEER

WOODPECKER

SALMON

BROWN BEAR

SOUTH: SUMMER

Stone affinity
Each birth time has a particular stone associated with it (see pp.14–15).

Tree affinity
Each birth time is connected to a type of tree (see pp.14–15).

Birth totem
An animal totem represents each birth time (see pp.16–17).

Directional totem
One of four cardinal Directions exerts an influence on each birth time (see pp.18–19).

Principal Element
Each birth time is fundamentally influenced by one of the four Elements (see pp.20–21).

Energy flow
Energy alternates between active and receptive with each birth time (see p.24).

Elemental Aspect
Each birth time has its own Elemental Aspect (see pp.20–21).

THE TWELVE
BIRTH TIMES

THE STRUCTURE OF THE MEDICINE WHEEL IS BASED
UPON THE SEASONS TO REFLECT THE POWERFUL
INFLUENCE OF NATURE ON HUMAN PERSONALITY.

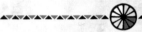

T he Medicine Wheel classifies human nature into twelve personality types, each corresponding to the characteristics of Nature at a particular time of the year. It is designed to act as a kind of map to help you discover your strengths and weaknesses, your inner drives and instinctive behaviours, and your true potential.

The four seasons form the basis of the Wheel's structure, with the Summer and Winter solstices and the Spring and Autumn equinoxes marking each season's passing. In Earth Medicine,

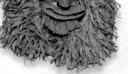

Seasonal rites
Performers at the Iroquois mid-Winter ceremony wore masks made of braided maize husks. They danced to attune themselves to energies that would ensure a good harvest.

each season is a metaphor for a stage of human growth and development. Spring is likened to infancy and the newness of life, and Summer to the exuberance of youth and of rapid development. Autumn represents the fulfilment that mature adulthood brings, while Winter symbolizes the accumulated wisdom that can be drawn upon in later life.

Each seasonal quarter of the Wheel is further divided into three periods, making twelve time segments altogether. The time of your birth determines the direction from which

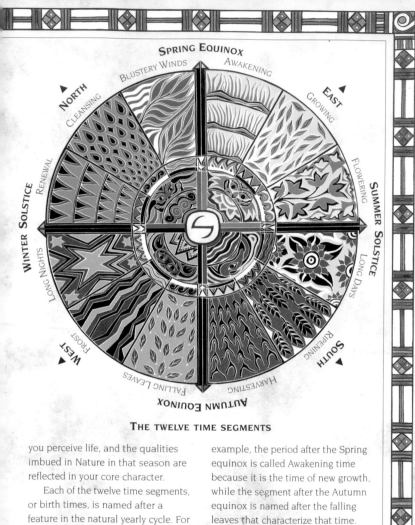

SPRING EQUINOX

BLUSTERY WINDS · AWAKENING

NORTH

CLEANSING · GROWING · **EAST**

RENEWAL · FLOWERING

WINTER SOLSTICE · **SUMMER SOLSTICE**

LONG NIGHTS · LONG DAYS

FROST · **WEST** · RIPENING · **SOUTH**

FALLING LEAVES · HARVESTING

AUTUMN EQUINOX

THE TWELVE TIME SEGMENTS

you perceive life, and the qualities imbued in Nature in that season are reflected in your core character.

Each of the twelve time segments, or birth times, is named after a feature in the natural yearly cycle. For

example, the period after the Spring equinox is called Awakening time because it is the time of new growth, while the segment after the Autumn equinox is named after the falling leaves that characterize that time.

THE SIGNIFICANCE OF
TOTEMS

NATIVE AMERICANS BELIEVED THAT TOTEMS — ANIMAL
SYMBOLS — REPRESENTED ESSENTIAL TRUTHS AND ACTED
AS CONNECTIONS TO NATURAL POWERS.

A totem is an animal or natural object adopted as an emblem to typify certain distinctive qualities. Native Americans regarded animals, whose behaviour is predictable, as particularly useful guides to categorizing human patterns of behaviour.

A totem mirrors aspects of your nature and unlocks the intuitive knowledge that lies beyond the reasoning capacity of the intellect. It may take the form of a carving or moulding, a pictorial image, or a token of fur, feather,

bone, tooth, or claw. Its presence serves as an immediate link with the energies it represents. A totem is therefore more effective than a glyph or symbol as an aid to comprehending non-physical powers and formative forces.

PRIMARY TOTEMS

In Earth Medicine you have three primary totems: a birth totem, a Directional totem, and an Elemental totem. Your *birth totem* is the embodiment of core characteristics that correspond with the dominant aspects of Nature during your birth time.

Symbol of strength
The handle of this Tlingit knife is carved with a raven and a bear head, symbols of insight and inner strength.

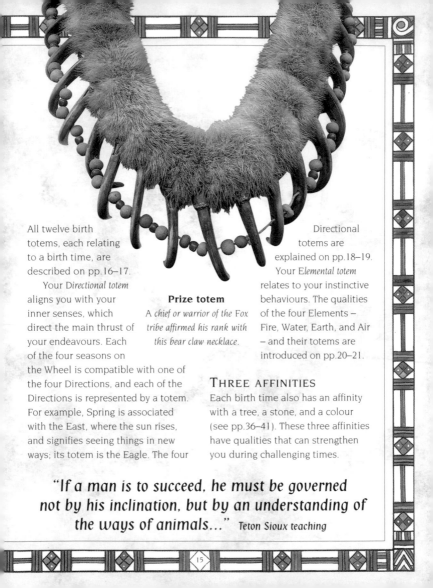

All twelve birth totems, each relating to a birth time, are described on pp.16–17.

Your *Directional totem* aligns you with your inner senses, which direct the main thrust of your endeavours. Each of the four seasons on the Wheel is compatible with one of the four Directions, and each of the Directions is represented by a totem. For example, Spring is associated with the East, where the sun rises, and signifies seeing things in new ways; its totem is the Eagle. The four

Prize totem
A chief or warrior of the Fox tribe affirmed his rank with this bear claw necklace.

Directional totems are explained on pp.18–19.

Your *Elemental totem* relates to your instinctive behaviours. The qualities of the four Elements – Fire, Water, Earth, and Air – and their totems are introduced on pp.20–21.

THREE AFFINITIES

Each birth time also has an affinity with a tree, a stone, and a colour (see pp.36–41). These three affinities have qualities that can strengthen you during challenging times.

"If a man is to succeed, he must be governed not by his inclination, but by an understanding of the ways of animals…" Teton Sioux teaching

THE TWELVE
BIRTH TOTEMS

THE TWELVE BIRTH TIMES ARE REPRESENTED BY TOTEMS,
EACH ONE AN ANIMAL THAT BEST EXPRESSES THE
QUALITIES INHERENT IN THAT BIRTH TIME.

Earth Medicine associates an animal totem with each birth time (the two sets of dates below reflect the difference in season between the northern and southern hemispheres). These animals help to connect you to the powers and abilities that they represent. For an in-depth study of the Goose birth totem, see pp.28–29.

FALCON
21 March–19 April (N. Hem)
22 Sept–22 Oct (S. Hem)
Falcons are full of initiative, but often rush in to make decisions they may later regret. Lively and extroverted, they have enthusiasm for new experiences but can sometimes lack persistence.

DEER
21 May–20 June (N. Hem)
23 Nov–21 Dec (S. Hem)
Deer are willing to sacrifice the old for the new. They loathe routine, thriving on variety and challenges. They have a wild side, often leaping from one situation or relationship into another without reflection.

BEAVER
20 April–20 May (N. Hem)
23 Oct–22 Nov (S. Hem)
Practical and steady, Beavers have a capacity for perseverance. Good homemakers, they are warm and affectionate but need harmony and peace to avoid becoming irritable. They have a keen aesthetic sense.

WOODPECKER
21 June–21 July (N. Hem)
22 Dec–19 Jan (S. Hem)
Emotional and sensitive, Woodpeckers are warm to those closest to them, and willing to sacrifice their needs for those of their loved ones. They have lively imaginations but can be worriers.

SALMON

22 July–21 August (N. Hem)
20 Jan–18 Feb (S. Hem)

Enthusiastic and self-confident,
Salmon people enjoy running things.
They are uncompromising and
forceful, and can occasionally seem a
little arrogant or self-important. They
are easily hurt by neglect.

BROWN BEAR

22 August–21 Sept (N. Hem)
19 Feb–20 March (S. Hem)

Brown Bears are hardworking,
practical, and self-reliant. They do
not like change, preferring to stick
to what is familiar. They have a flair
for fixing things, are good-natured,
and make good friends.

CROW

22 Sept–22 Oct (N. Hem)
21 March–19 April (S. Hem)

Crows dislike solitude and feel most
comfortable in company. Although
usually pleasant and good-natured,
they can be strongly influenced by
negative atmospheres, becoming
gloomy and prickly.

SNAKE

23 Oct–22 Nov (N. Hem)
20 April–20 May (S. Hem)

Snakes are secretive and
mysterious, hiding their feelings
beneath a cool exterior. Adaptable,
determined, and imaginative, they
are capable of bouncing back from
tough situations encountered in life.

OWL

23 Nov–21 Dec (N. Hem)
21 May–20 June (S. Hem)

Owls need freedom of expression.
They are lively, self-reliant, and have
an eye for detail. Inquisitive and
adaptable, they have a tendency to
overextend themselves. Owls are
often physically courageous.

GOOSE

22 Dec–19 Jan (N. Hem)
21 June–21 July (S. Hem)

Goose people are far-sighted
idealists who are willing to explore
the unknown. They approach life with
enthusiasm, determined to fulfil their
dreams. They are perfectionists, and
can appear unduly serious.

OTTER

20 Jan–18 Feb (N. Hem)
22 July–21 August (S. Hem)

Otters are friendly, lively, and
perceptive. They feel inhibited by
too many rules and regulations,
which often makes them appear
eccentric. They like cleanliness and
order, and have original minds.

WOLF

19 Feb–20 March (N. Hem)
22 August–21 Sept (S. Hem)

Wolves are sensitive, artistic, and
intuitive – people to whom others
turn for help. They value freedom
and their own space, and are easily
affected by others. They are
philosophical, trusting, and genuine.

THE INFLUENCE OF THE
DIRECTIONS

ALSO KNOWN BY NATIVE AMERICANS AS THE FOUR WINDS, THE INFLUENCE OF THE FOUR DIRECTIONS IS EXPERIENCED THROUGH YOUR INNER SENSES.

Regarded as the "keepers" or "caretakers" of the Universe, the four Directions or alignments were also referred to by Native Americans as the four Winds because their presence was felt rather than seen.

DIRECTIONAL TOTEMS

In Earth Medicine, each Direction or Wind is associated with a season and a time of day. Thus the Winter birth times – Renewal time, Cleansing time, and Blustery Winds time –

all fall within the North Direction, and night. The Direction to which your birth time belongs influences the nature of your inner senses.

The East Direction is associated with illumination. Its totem is the Eagle – a bird that soars close to the Sun and can see clearly from height. The South is the Direction of Summer and the afternoon. It signifies growth and fruition, fluidity, and emotions. Its totem, the Mouse, symbolizes productivity, feelings, and an ability to perceive detail.

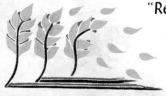

"Remember...the circle of the sky, the stars, the super-natural Winds breathing night and day...the four Directions." Pawnee teaching

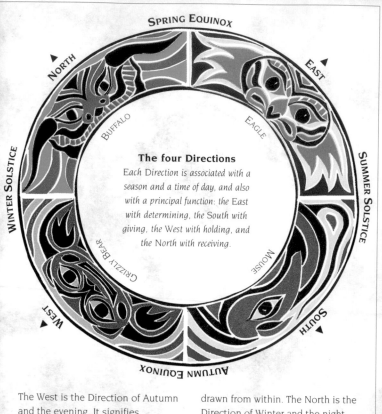

The four Directions

Each Direction is associated with a season and a time of day, and also with a principal function: the East with determining, the South with giving, the West with holding, and the North with receiving.

SPRING EQUINOX

NORTH

EAST

WINTER SOLSTICE

SUMMER SOLSTICE

BUFFALO

EAGLE

GRIZZLY BEAR

MOUSE

WEST

SOUTH

AUTUMN EQUINOX

The West is the Direction of Autumn and the evening. It signifies transformation – from day to night, from Summer to Winter – and the qualities of introspection and conservation. Its totem is the Grizzly Bear, which represents strength

drawn from within. The North is the Direction of Winter and the night, and is associated with the mind and its sustenance – knowledge. Its totem is the Buffalo, an animal that was honoured by Native Americans as the great material "provider".

THE INFLUENCE OF THE ELEMENTS

THE FOUR ELEMENTS – AIR, FIRE, WATER, AND EARTH –
PERVADE EVERYTHING AND INDICATE THE NATURE OF
MOVEMENT AND THE ESSENCE OF WHO YOU ARE.

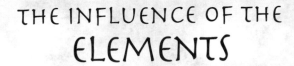

Elements are intangible qualities
that describe the essential state
or character of all things. In
Earth Medicine, the four Elements
are allied with four fundamental modes
of activity and are associated with
different aspects of the self. Air
expresses free movement in all
directions; it is related to the
mind and to thinking. Fire
indicates expansive
motion; it is linked with
the spirit and with
intuition. Water
signifies fluidity; it

Elemental profile
*The Elemental config-
uration of Goose is Earth
of Air. Air is the Principal
Element and Earth the
Elemental Aspect.*

WATER

AIR

EARTH

FIRE

AIR

EARTH

has associations with the soul and the emotions. Earth symbolizes stability; it is related to the physical body and the sensations.

ELEMENTAL DISTRIBUTION

On the Medicine Wheel one Element is associated with each of the four Directions – Fire in the East, Earth in the West, Air in the North, and Water in the South. These are known as the Principal Elements.

The four Elements also have an individual association with each of the twelve birth times – known as the Elemental Aspects. They follow a cyclical sequence around the Wheel based on the action of the Sun (Fire) on the Earth, producing atmosphere (Air) and condensation (Water).

The three birth times that share an Elemental Aspect belong to the same Elemental family or "clan", with a totem that gives insight into its key characteristics. Goose people belong to the Turtle clan (see pp.34–35).

ELEMENTAL EMPHASIS

For each birth time, the qualities of the Elemental Aspect usually predominate over those of the Principal Element, although both are present to give a specific configuration, such as Fire of Earth (for Goose's, see pp.34–35). For Falcon, Wood-pecker, and Otter, the Principal Element and the Elemental Aspect are identical (for example, Air of Air), so people of these totems tend to express that Element intensely.

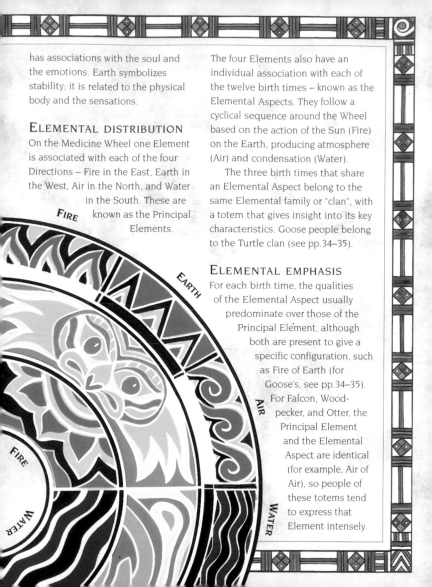

FIRE

EARTH

AIR

FIRE

WATER

WATER

THE INFLUENCE OF THE MOON

THE WAXING AND WANING OF THE MOON DURING ITS
FOUR PHASES HAS A CRUCIAL INFLUENCE ON THE
FORMATION OF PERSONALITY AND HUMAN ENDEAVOUR.

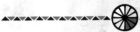

Native Americans regarded the Sun and Moon as indicators respectively of the active and receptive energies inherent in Nature (see p.24), as well as the measurers of time. They associated solar influences with conscious activity and the exercise of reason and the will, and lunar influences with subconscious activity and the emotional and intuitive aspects of human nature.

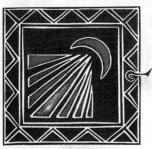

The Waxing Moon

This phase lasts for approximately eleven days. It is a time of growth and therefore ideal for developing new ideas and concentrating your efforts into new projects.

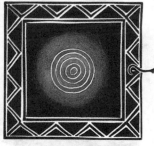

The Full Moon

Lasting about three days, this is when lunar power is at its height. It is therefore a good time for completing what was developed during the Waxing Moon.

THE FOUR PHASES

There are four phases in the twenty-nine-day lunar cycle, each one an expression of energy reflecting a particular mode of activity. They can be likened to the phases of growth of a flowering plant through the seasons: the emergence of buds (Waxing Moon), the bursting of flowers (Full Moon), the falling away of flowers (Waning Moon), and the germination of seeds (Dark Moon). The influence of each phase can be felt in two ways: in the formation of personality and in day-to-day life.

The energy expressed by the phase of the Moon at the time of your birth has a strong influence on personality. For instance, someone born during the Dark Moon is likely to be inward-looking, whilst a person born during the Full Moon may be more expressive. Someone born during a Waxing Moon is likely to have an outgoing nature, whilst a person born during a Waning Moon may be reserved. Consult a set of Moon tables to discover the phase the Moon was in on *your* birthday.

In your day-to-day life, the benefits of coming into harmony with the Moon's energies are considerable. Experience the energy of the four phases by consciously working with them. A Native American approach is described below.

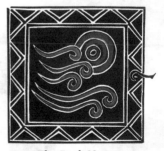

The Waning Moon

A time for making changes, this phase lasts for an average of eleven days. Use it to improve and modify, and to dispose of what is no longer needed or wanted.

The Dark Moon

The Moon disappears from the sky for around four days. This is a time for contemplation of what has been achieved, and for germinating the seeds for the new.

THE INFLUENCE OF
ENERGY FLOW

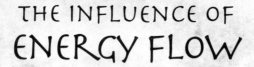

THE MEDICINE WHEEL REFLECTS THE PERFECT
BALANCE OF THE COMPLEMENTARY ACTIVE AND
RECEPTIVE ENERGIES THAT CO-EXIST IN NATURE.

Energy flows through Nature in two complementary ways, which can be expressed in terms of active and receptive, or male and female. The active energy principle is linked with the Elements of Fire and Air, and the receptive principle with Water and Earth.

Each of the twelve birth times has an active or receptive energy related to its Elemental Aspect. Travelling around the Wheel, the two energies alternate with each birth time, resulting in an equal balance of active and receptive energies, as in Nature.

Active energy is associated with the Sun and conscious activity. Those whose birth times take this principle prefer to pursue experience. They are conceptual,

energetic, outgoing, practical, and analytical. Receptive energy is associated with the Moon and subconscious activity. Those whose birth times take this principle prefer to attract experience. They are intuitive, reflective, conserving, emotional, and nurturing.

THE WAKAN-TANKA

At the heart of the Wheel lies an S-shape within a circle, the symbol of the life-giving source of everything that comes into physical existence – seemingly out of nothing. Named by the Plains Indians as Wakan-Tanka (Great Power), it can also be perceived as energy coming into form and form reverting to energy in the unending continuity of life.

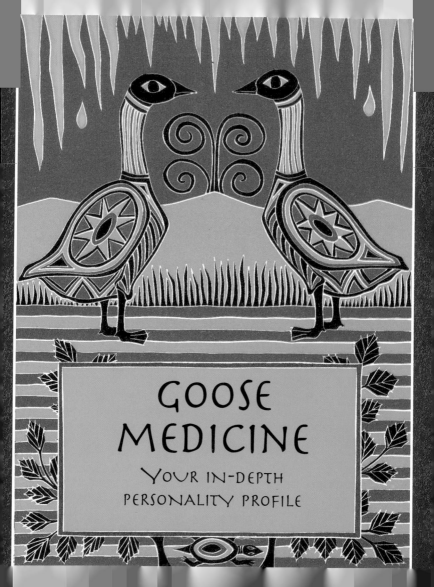

GOOSE
MEDICINE

YOUR IN-DEPTH
PERSONALITY PROFILE

SEASON OF BIRTH
RENEWAL TIME

THE AUSTERE NATURE OF WINTER BEGINS IN THE FIRST
BIRTH TIME OF THE SEASON, LENDING THOSE BORN THEN
THE QUALITIES OF SELF-SUFFICIENCY AND PATIENCE.

Renewal time is one of the twelve birth times, the fundamental division of the year into twelve seasonal segments (see pp.12–13). As the first period of the Winter cycle, it is the time of year when the wind is cold and piercing and the Earth barren. Yet it is also a time of hope as the days begin to lengthen, heralding the start of a new yearly cycle.

just as the Earth lies dormant beneath the hard and frozen surface of the soil, waiting to burst into life with the arrival of the warm, Spring days, so, if you were born during Renewal time, you possess patience and faith that your hopes and ambitions will eventually reach fruition.

During this season all human and animal life withdraws as much as possible from outdoor activities, seeking shelter from the harsh environment. This is reflected in your own reserved, inward-looking, and thoughtful nature, and in your self-sufficient approach to life.

INFLUENCE OF NATURE
The qualities and characteristics imbued in Nature at this time form the basis of your own nature. So,

Traditionally, the Pueblo peoples marked the beginning of this period with the buffalo dance. This ceremony was perfomed to drive away sickness and disease, and to bring purifying snows. It also celebrated the renewal or purification of mind and body, which emerged after the dance refreshed and energized.

STAGE OF LIFE

This time of year might be compared to the maturity and confidence experienced as the middle years of life come to a close. In human development terms, it is a period in which a high degree of self-confidence, stability, and security has been achieved. In consequence, it is a time of increased freedom of mind, body, and spirit, resulting in fresh ideas and new ways of being.

ACHIEVE YOUR POTENTIAL

You have clear, long-term aspirations and the patience and determination to achieve them even when the circumstances appear adverse. However, although you generally accept disappointments with

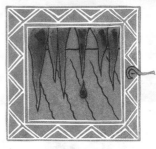

Nature's energy

Nature begins its most austere phase in this, the first cycle of Winter after the Winter solstice. Cold, biting winds attempt to penetrate the frozen, barren Earth, purifying and renewing everything in their path.

fortitude, beware of sinking into despondency and melancholy when faced with continued frustration of the achievement of your goals, as you may become embittered.

Your single-mindedness, together with your natural reserve, can make you appear cool and aloof to those you actually hold dear. Try to reveal the gentleness of your heart by expressing more often, in both word and deed, the tenderness you feel towards them.

"Life is a circle from childhood to childhood; so it is with everything where power moves." Black Elk teaching

BIRTH TOTEM
THE GOOSE

THE ESSENTIAL NATURE AND CHARACTERISTIC
BEHAVIOUR OF THE GOOSE EXPRESSES THE PERSONALITY
TYPE OF THOSE BORN DURING RENEWAL TIME.

Like the goose, people born during Renewal time are purposeful, far-sighted, and resourceful. If you were born at this time, you have an ambitious, steadfast, and imaginative nature that thrives on the freedom to reach for the stars.

Imaginative and determined, you seek the fulfilment of your dreams and aspirations with purpose and vigour. Single-minded and resourceful, you pursue distant goals with enthusiasm, willing to forego many of life's pleasures and suffer temporary hardships in order to fulfil your objectives.

Goose power
Determined and aspirational, the goose also expresses the single-minded and imaginative aspects of the purposeful, trustworthy, and reserved people born at this time.

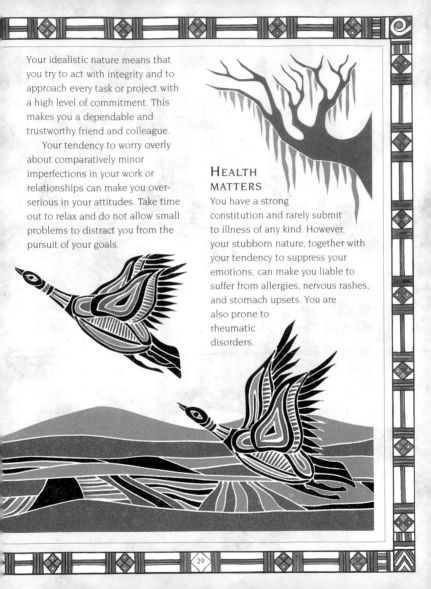

Your idealistic nature means that you try to act with integrity and to approach every task or project with a high level of commitment. This makes you a dependable and trustworthy friend and colleague.

Your tendency to worry overly about comparatively minor imperfections in your work or relationships can make you over-serious in your attitudes. Take time out to relax and do not allow small problems to distract you from the pursuit of your goals.

HEALTH MATTERS

You have a strong constitution and rarely submit to illness of any kind. However, your stubborn nature, together with your tendency to suppress your emotions, can make you liable to suffer from allergies, nervous rashes, and stomach upsets. You are also prone to rheumatic disorders.

THE GOOSE AND
RELATIONSHIPS

RESOURCEFUL, AMBITIOUS GOOSE PEOPLE MAKE
DEPENDABLE FRIENDS. THEY ARE FAITHFUL AND
COMMITTED PARTNERS BUT OFTEN HIDE THEIR FEELINGS.

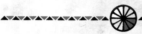

Far-sighted Goose people, like their totem animal, pursue distant goals with energy. If your birth totem is Goose, your ambitious and determined nature may inspire others, but it excites admiration and respect more often than affection. At times aloof, you are very self-reliant and prefer not to be over-involved with others, though you may let one or two people close to your tender heart. You tend to be over-serious; try to learn to let go – you'll be surprised how much fun you can have.

LOVING RELATIONSHIPS

Goose people crave the protection and security of a lasting relationship. They rarely fall in love at first sight, but, once captured, should remain true and devoted. Male Goose is

trustworthy and dependable, while female Goose is energetic and a first-rate home-maker. Both rarely show affection in public, but they can be deeply sensual lovers in private.

When problems arise, it is often because you hide your feelings with a mask of cool independence. Showing your more vulnerable side will forge a greater bond of intimacy and trust with your partner.

COPING WITH GOOSE

Goose people are practical realists, so adopt a down-to-earth approach as they rarely respond to emotional appeals. They dislike the merest hint of insincerity: be true and straight with them to make headway. Their perfectionist nature may seem demanding, but in fact they are always hardest on themselves.

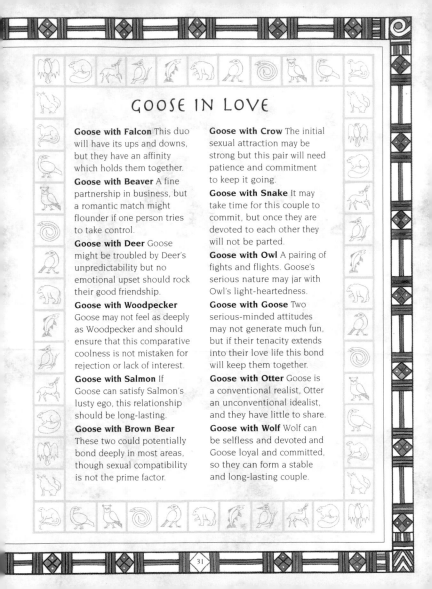

GOOSE IN LOVE

Goose with Falcon This duo will have its ups and downs, but they have an affinity which holds them together.

Goose with Beaver A fine partnership in business, but a romantic match might flounder if one person tries to take control.

Goose with Deer Goose might be troubled by Deer's unpredictability but no emotional upset should rock their good friendship.

Goose with Woodpecker Goose may not feel as deeply as Woodpecker and should ensure that this comparative coolness is not mistaken for rejection or lack of interest.

Goose with Salmon If Goose can satisfy Salmon's lusty ego, this relationship should be long-lasting.

Goose with Brown Bear These two could potentially bond deeply in most areas, though sexual compatibility is not the prime factor.

Goose with Crow The initial sexual attraction may be strong but this pair will need patience and commitment to keep it going.

Goose with Snake It may take time for this couple to commit, but once they are devoted to each other they will not be parted.

Goose with Owl A pairing of fights and flights. Goose's serious nature may jar with Owl's light-heartedness.

Goose with Goose Two serious-minded attitudes may not generate much fun, but if their tenacity extends into their love life this bond will keep them together.

Goose with Otter Goose is a conventional realist, Otter an unconventional idealist, and they have little to share.

Goose with Wolf Wolf can be selfless and devoted and Goose loyal and committed, so they can form a stable and long-lasting couple.

DIRECTIONAL TOTEM
THE BUFFALO

THE BUFFALO SYMBOLIZES THE INFLUENCE OF THE
NORTH ON GOOSE PEOPLE, WHOSE PATIENCE AND PURITY
OF PURPOSE ENABLES THEM TO ACHIEVE THEIR GOALS.

Renewal time, Cleansing time, and Blustery Winds time all fall within the quarter of the Medicine Wheel associated with the North Direction or Wind.

The North is aligned with Winter and with night, and it is therefore associated with patience, the hidden energy that lies beneath the surface, purity, and renewal. It is likened to the preparation for new life and new ideas – the reflective stillness that precedes rebirth and the time of rapid growth. The power of the North's influence is primarily with the mind and wisdom, and its principal function is the power of sustenance. It takes as its totem the revered and life-sustaining buffalo.

Buffalo skull
This Blackfeet-painted buffalo skull represents the buffalo, which is associated with sustenance of mind and body.

The specific influence of the North on Goose people is on purity of intent and purpose, bringing the apparently impossible within reach. It is associated with renewal of both mind and body, such as you feel the moment you awake after a refreshing sleep, bringing strength, wisdom, and patience for the attainment of your dreams.

BUFFALO CHARACTERISTICS
Of all animals, the buffalo was most revered by Native Americans because many tribes depended on it for their survival. Every part of it was

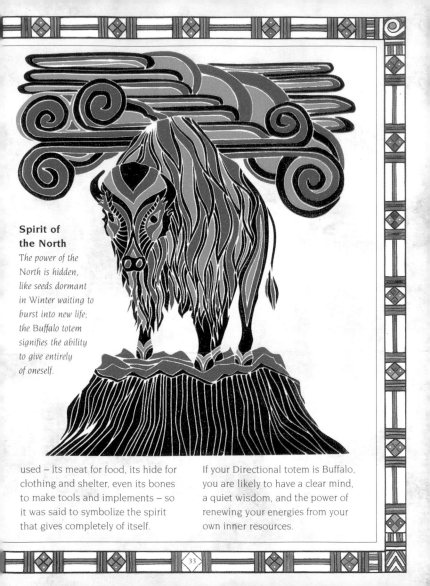

Spirit of the North

The power of the North is hidden, like seeds dormant in Winter waiting to burst into new life; the Buffalo totem signifies the ability to give entirely of oneself.

used – its meat for food, its hide for clothing and shelter, even its bones to make tools and implements – so it was said to symbolize the spirit that gives completely of itself.

If your Directional totem is Buffalo, you are likely to have a clear mind, a quiet wisdom, and the power of renewing your energies from your own inner resources.

ELEMENTAL TOTEM
THE TURTLE

LIKE THE TURTLE, WHICH TAKES LIFE ONE STEP AT A TIME, GOOSE PEOPLE'S PERSISTENT NATURE MEANS THEY ARE PATIENT IN THE PURSUIT OF THEIR GOALS.

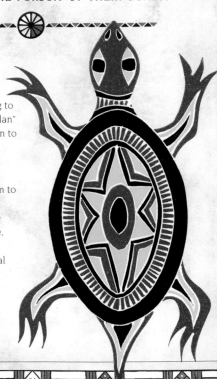

The Elemental Aspect of Goose people is Earth. They share this Aspect with Beaver and Brown Bear people, who all therefore belong to the same Elemental family or "clan" (see pp.20–21 for an introduction to the influence of the Elements).

THE TURTLE CLAN

Each Elemental clan has a totem to provide insight into its essential characteristics. The totem of the Elemental clan of Earth is Turtle, which symbolizes a persistent, careful, practical, and methodical nature with a mature outlook.

Down to Earth
The turtle symbolizes the fundamental qualities of the Element of Earth: stability and persistence.

The turtle is a gentle creature, working steadily towards its desired destination at its own pace. So, if you belong to this clan, you will have a patient, down-to-earth personality and be tenacious about your goals.

Constructive and creative, you will work hard and overcome obstacles to achieve results. You dislike disorder and feel threatened by change. You can be inflexible, and crave stability in order to feel at ease.

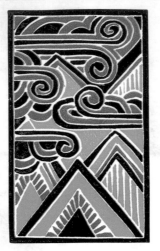

Earth of Air

The Element of Earth feeds Air, generating a capacity for steadiness and strong idealism.

idealistic power of Air. So you may sometimes lose sight of the lighter pleasures of life and become anxious about minor matters. This can make you tense and moody and you may feel misunderstood by other people.

ELEMENTAL PROFILE

For Goose people, the predominant Elemental Aspect of persistent Earth is fundamentally affected by the qualities of your Principal Element – invigorating Air. Consequently, if you were born at this time you are likely to be persevering and dependable with a lively mind, which is bent on effecting change.

You may have a tendency to be over-serious, driven by the heavy solidity of Earth, and the intellectual,

At times like these, or when you are feeling low or lacking in energy, try the following revitalizing exercise. Find a quiet spot in a woodland, park, or garden, away from the polluting effects of traffic and the activities of others.

You have an instinctive affinity for the Earth and plants, so sit or stand with both feet firmly in contact with the ground, and simply notice and receive the natural beauty of growing things around you. Breathe slowly and deeply, allowing the energizing power of the life-force to refresh your body, mind, and spirit.

STONE AFFINITY
PERIDOT

BY USING THE GEMSTONE WITH WHICH YOUR OWN ESSENCE RESONATES, YOU CAN TAP INTO THE POWER OF THE EARTH ITSELF AND AWAKEN YOUR INNER STRENGTHS.

Gemstones are minerals that are formed within the Earth itself in a very slow but continuous process. Native Americans valued them not only for their beauty but also for being literally part of the Earth, and therefore possessing part of its life-force. They regarded gemstones as being "alive" – channellers of energy that could be used in many ways: to heal, to protect, or for meditation.

Every gemstone has a different energy or vibration. On the Medicine Wheel, a stone is associated with each birth time, the energy of which resonates with the essence of those

Faceted peridot
Regarded as "petrified" heavenly radiance, peridot is related to clear-sightedness and clarity of mind.

born during that time. Because of this energy affiliation, your gemstone can be used to help bring you into harmony with the Earth and to create balance within yourself. It can enhance and develop your good qualities and endow you with the qualities or abilities you need.

ENERGY RESONANCE

Goose people have an affinity with peridot, a gem-quality form of the mineral olivine. It is bottle-green in colour and has a characteristic oily sheen. Believed to impart spiritual strength, peridot is associated with intuitive insight and inner vision.

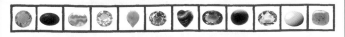

ACTIVATE YOUR GEMSTONE

O btain a piece of peridot and cleanse it by holding it under cold running water. Allow it to dry naturally, then, holding the stone with both hands, bring it up to your mouth and blow into it sharply and hard three or four times in order to impregnate it with your breath. Next, hold it firmly in one hand and silently welcome it into your life as a friend and helper.

When you have a choice to make or a challenge ahead, use the peridot to help you meditate on the issue. Find a quiet spot to sit without fear of interruption and hold the stone in your left hand to receive its subtle energies. Focus on the problem and, with the help of your stone, seek guidance on the path to follow. Listen for the still, small voice of your inner self.

Native Americans likened it to a spiritual Sun and its radiance was thought to impart clarity, helping you recognize the true meaning of any changes taking place in your life. It was also used to help recover lost or mislaid items.

If your birth totem is Goose, peridot can be useful in replenishing your innate reserves of inner strength and

in lending your natural foresight the depth of intuitive wisdom. It also has a soothing energy, so it can offer comfort at times when you feel pessimistic, tense, or misunderstood.

Peridot power
To benefit most from its effect, wear peridot in a ring, or at the base of the throat in a necklace.

"The outline of the stone is round; the power of the stone is endless." *Lakota Sioux teaching*

TREE AFFINITY
SILVER BIRCH

GAIN A DEEPER UNDERSTANDING OF YOUR OWN NATURE
AND AWAKEN POWERS LYING DORMANT WITHIN YOU BY
RESPECTING AND CONNECTING WITH YOUR AFFINITY TREE.

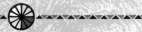

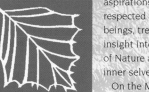

Trees have an important part to play in the protection of Nature's mechanisms and in the maintenance of the Earth's atmospheric balance, which is essential for the survival of the human race.

Native Americans referred to trees as "Standing People" because they stand firm, obtaining strength from their connection with the Earth. They therefore teach us the importance of being grounded, whilst at the same time listening to, and reaching for, our higher aspirations. When respected as living beings, trees can provide insight into the workings of Nature and our own inner selves.

On the Medicine Wheel, each birth time is associated with a particular kind of tree, the basic qualities of which complement the nature of those born during that time. Goose people have an affinity with the silver birch. With its strikingly white bark, this tree symbolizes purity of motive and clarity of intent – both essential aspects of the Goose personality.

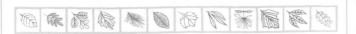

CONNECT WITH YOUR TREE

Appreciate the beauty of your affinity tree and study its nature carefully, for it has an affinity with your own nature.

The silver birch is a slender and graceful tree with silver-white, peeling bark, and delicate, light green, pointed leaves. Its timber was once valued for making boats and cradles, while the bark has been used for writing on instead of paper.

Try the following exercise when you need to revitalize your inner strength. Stand beside your affinity tree. Place the palms of your hands on its trunk and rest your forehead on the backs of your hands. Inhale slowly and experience energy from the tree's roots flow through your body. If easily available, obtain a cutting or twig from your affinity tree to keep as a totem or helper.

The silver birch is also associated with childhood and protection. At times, strict adherence to their ideals makes Goose people take life rather too seriously. At such times, they tap into the child within themselves by connecting with their tree (see panel above).

LETTING GO

If your birth totem is Goose, you are resourceful and single-minded but can be reserved and too inward-looking. This, along with your high principles, can make you seem aloof, keeping other people at a distance.

Just as the silver birch lets its outer bark peel away, revealing the layer beneath, so you can learn to let go and allow those close to you to see your inner nature and your gentle heart. Call on the silver birch and draw on its bright, uplifting energy to raise your spirits when you feel despondent and inspire you to relax and enjoy greater freedom.

"All healing plants are given by Wakan-Tanka; therefore they are holy." Lakota Sioux teaching

COLOUR AFFINITY
WHITE

Enhance your positive qualities by using the
power of your affinity colour to affect your
emotional and mental states.

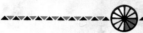

Each birth time has an affinity with a particular colour. This is the colour that resonates best with the energies of the people born during that time. Exposure to your affinity colour will encourage a positive emotional and mental outlook, while exposure to colours that clash with your affinity colour will have a negative effect on your sense of well-being.

White resonates with Goose people. Associated with purity and cleanliness, white is the colour of clarity of thought and penetrating insights. It suggests idealism and far-sighted or visionary abilities. It is an optimistic colour that enables you to focus on creative solutions to obstacles that may stand before you, or to embark on a fresh new path or direction if necessary. White

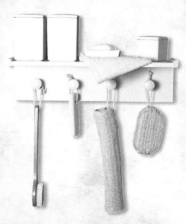

Colour scheme

Experience the full benefit of your colour affinity. Let a white colour theme be the thread that runs through your home, from the ornaments to the fixtures and fittings.

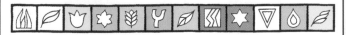

MEDITATE ON YOUR COLOUR

Place some white flowers – lilies narcissi, chrysanthemums, roses – in a white vase. Take the vase to a room in which you will not be disturbed for at least half an hour and place the vase on a table. Sit at the table and face the flowers.

Focus all your attention on the white blooms. Relax your body and concentrate your mind on the colour. This will help you to clear your mind of distractions. Feel the colour energizing every cell of your body. If a difficult situation or problem confronts you at the moment, meditate upon it. Allow any thoughts and sensations to flow through your mind and body, and reflect on them.

embodies high moral values and a sense of hope in times of difficulty, stimulating the determination needed to see a situation through to its satisfactory conclusion.

COLOUR BENEFITS

Strengthen your aura and enhance your positive qualities by introducing white – or shades of off-white – to the interior decor of your home. Touches of white can make all the difference. A white lampshade or clear white spotlights, for example, can alter the ambience of a room, or try diffusing natural light by replacing curtains with white Japanese paper blinds.

If you need a confidence boost, wear something that contains white. Whenever your energies are low, practise the colour meditation exercise outlined above to balance your emotions, awaken your creativity, and help you feel joyful.

"The power of the spirit should be honoured with its colour." Lakota Sioux teaching

WORKING THE WHEEL
LIFE PATH

CONSIDER YOUR BIRTH PROFILE AS A STARTING POINT IN
THE DEVELOPMENT OF YOUR CHARACTER AND THE
ACHIEVEMENT OF PERSONAL FULFILMENT.

Each of the twelve birth times is associated with a particular path of learning, or with a collection of lessons to be learned through life. By following your path of learning you will develop strengths in place of weaknesses, achieve a greater sense of harmony with the world, and discover inner peace.

YOUR PATH OF LEARNING
For Goose people, the first lesson on your path of learning is to cultivate the

ability to complete projects. By nature perfectionist and pessimistic, you tend to see major problems where in fact only minor ones exist, allowing them to impede your progress unnecessarily. Try not to let minor imperfections prevent the development of an otherwise excellent idea or scheme. Try to keep problems in perspective, and focus your mind on the achievement of

"Each man's road is shown to him within his own heart. There he sees all the truths of life." Cheyenne teaching

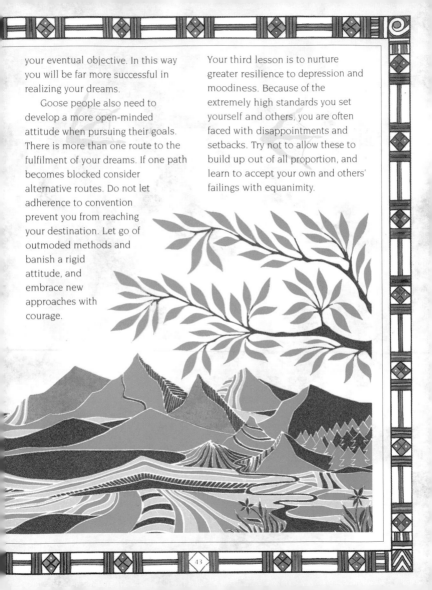

your eventual objective. In this way you will be far more successful in realizing your dreams.

Goose people also need to develop a more open-minded attitude when pursuing their goals. There is more than one route to the fulfilment of your dreams. If one path becomes blocked consider alternative routes. Do not let adherence to convention prevent you from reaching your destination. Let go of outmoded methods and banish a rigid attitude, and embrace new approaches with courage.

Your third lesson is to nurture greater resilience to depression and moodiness. Because of the extremely high standards you set yourself and others, you are often faced with disappointments and setbacks. Try not to allow these to build up out of all proportion, and learn to accept your own and others' failings with equanimity.

WORKING THE WHEEL
MEDICINE POWER

HARNESS THE POWERS OF OTHER BIRTH TIMES TO
TRANSFORM YOUR WEAKNESSES INTO STRENGTHS AND
MEET THE CHALLENGES IN YOUR LIFE.

The whole spectrum of human qualities and abilities is represented on the Medicine Wheel. The totems and affinities associated with each birth time indicate the basic qualities with which those born at that time are equipped.

Study your path of learning (see pp.42–43) to identify those aspects of your personality that may need to be strengthened, then look at other birth times to discover the totems and affinities that can assist you in this task. For example, your Elemental profile is Earth of Air (see pp.34–35); so for balance you need the adaptive qualities of Water and

Complementary affinity
A key strength of Woodpecker – weak in Goose – is the ability to act according to your heart.

the enthusiasm of Fire. Salmon's Elemental profile is Fire of Water and Woodpecker's is Water of Water, so meditate on these birth totems. In addition, you may find it useful to study the profiles of the other two members of your Elemental clan of Turtle – Beaver and Brown Bear – to discover how the same Elemental Aspect can be expressed differently.

Also helpful is the birth totem that sits opposite yours on the Medicine Wheel, which contains qualities and characteristics that complement or enhance your own. This is known as your complementary affinity, which for Goose people is Woodpecker.

ESSENTIAL STRENGTHS

D escribed below are the essential strengths of each birth totem. To develop a quality that is weak in yourself or that you need to meet a particular challenge, meditate upon the birth totem that contains the attribute you need. Obtain a representation of the relevant totem – a claw, tooth, or feather; a picture, ring, or model. Affirm that the power it represents is within you.

Falcon medicine is the power of keen observation and the ability to act decisively and energetically whenever action is required.

Beaver medicine is the ability to think creatively and laterally – to develop alternative ways of doing or thinking about things.

Deer medicine is characterized by sensitivity to the intentions of others and to that which might be detrimental to your well-being.

Woodpecker medicine is the ability to establish a steady rhythm throughout life and to be tenacious in protecting all that you hold dear.

Salmon medicine is the strength to be determined and courageous in the choice of goals you want to achieve and to have enough stamina to see a task through to the end.

Brown Bear medicine is the ability to be resourceful, hardworking, and dependable in times of need, and to draw on inner strength.

Crow medicine is the ability to transform negative or non-productive situations into positive ones and to transcend limitations.

Snake medicine is the talent to adapt easily to changes in circumstances and to manage transitional phases well.

Owl medicine is the power to see clearly during times of uncertainty and to conduct life consistently, according to long-term plans.

Goose medicine is the courage to do whatever might be necessary to protect your ideals and adhere to your principles in life.

Otter medicine is the ability to connect with your inner child, to be innovative and idealistic, and to thoroughly enjoy the ordinary tasks and routines of everyday life.

Wolf medicine is the courage to act according to your intuition and instincts rather than your intellect, and to be compassionate.

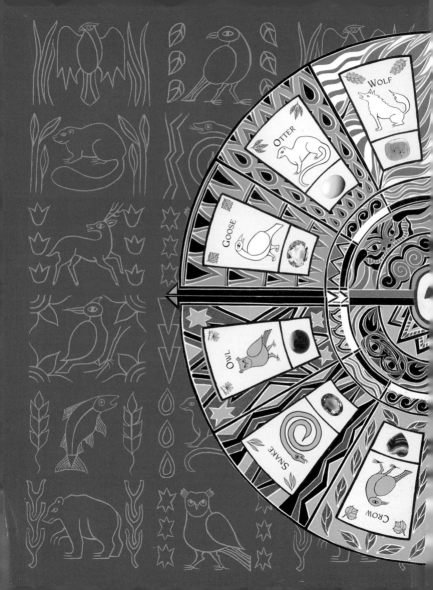